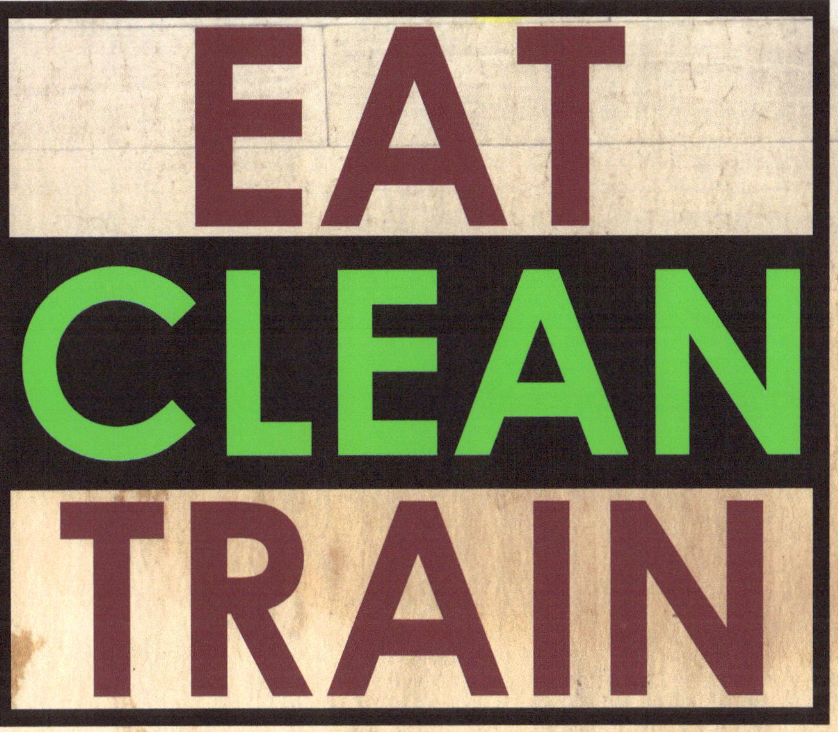

21 Day Guide To a Better Life

Created by: Ms. Gina Mondesir

Table of Contents

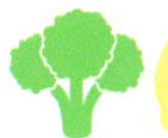

DISCLAIMER

The author, Gina Mondesir, is not a doctor. Before you participate in the 21 DAYS TO A BETTER LIFE, please consult with your primary doctor or physician.

The following document has been copy written and cannot be reproduce or distributed to other parties without the author consent.

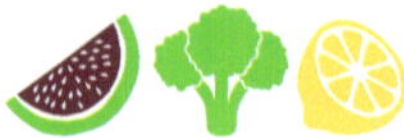

THE STARTING LINE

"It's never too late - never too late to start over, never too late to be happy."- Jane Fonda

YOU DID IT! Congratulations on taking the first step to gaining back the control of your body. It is true what they say, "Your body is a temple." By supplying your temple with healthy and rich foods, you are well on your way to a long lasting vibrant life.

PSA: THIS IS NOT A DIET. One word I loathe more than anything in the world is the word diet. The first three letters in diet is enough to make you jump off a cliff. We are not dying to live. I know there are a million and one diet pills, detox teas, or other fads out there. It almost feels like a diet devil vortex that is ready to suck you in at anytime.

However, this is a lifestyle. It is really that simple. In order for you to create the change you wish to see in yourself; you have to embrace this healthy mindset. You have to believe that this way of life is the greatest thing for you, your family, your kids, your spouse, or whoever loves to see you.

In the next 21 days you are reprogramming your body to desire a healthier way of living. Why 21 days?

"We are what we repeatedly do. Excellence, then, is not an act, but a habit." –Aristotle

Over the course of 21 days you are forming new patterns. Furthermore, it will only then become a habit if you make it a lifestyle.

Detoxification is the primary step to weight lost. One of the main reasons people struggle with losing weight is because their bodies are filled with loads of toxins. The toxins can be in the form of refined sugars, fried foods, processed foods, meats, refined carbohydrate, dairy, liquor, sodas, or other sugary drinks. This is how fat get stored. If your body is constantly overloaded with these toxins, it will not have the strength or energy to burn these calories.

Additionally, supplying your body with the wrong foods can lead to other complications as well. For instances diabetes, hypertension, bloating, acne, stress, insomnia, low sex drive, fatigue, or infertility can be a result of bad eating habits.

One of my reasons for embracing a healthier way of life is because I wanted to have a baby. My husband had a child prior to our relationship, so I had proof that he can conceive, but I didn't know if I could. This led me to research natural ways to prepare the womb for pregnancy. In my discovery, all I kept seeing with each article, video, or book is mainly that proper food and exercise can increase the chances of pregnancy.

Following this advice, it took me 6 months to conceive. Nevertheless, after conceiving, I was faced with a new challenge. My first doctor's appointment, I found out that I had fibroids. Obviously I was freaking out. My stress levels sky rocketed. I didn't even know what the heck fibroids were.

[Medical News Today](#) reports, *"**Uterine fibroids are non-cancerous tumors that grow from the muscle layers of the womb. These benign growths of smooth muscle can vary from the size of a bean to being as large as a melon.**"*

Although my husband and I planned to have a home-birth, my doctor didn't think it was possible considering my condition. She didn't even know how we were able to conceive. I had a total of 5 fibroids. She actually told me that fibroids are more common for women of color than any other race. So I indulge myself into more books. This time, the research was on fibroids and how to shrink them.

According to an article on draxe.com, *"**High-fat,** [processed meats](#) **are some of the worst food choices for women when it comes to fibroids. Foods high in unhealthy fats, like non-organic/processed meats or trans-fats (think hamburgers and processed breakfast sausages), can increase inflammation levels. Processed foods also often contain chemical additives and other ingredients that promote inflammation**."* Even though I was not consuming meat, I was still taking in a lot of process foods at that time. I knew I had to make a drastic change.

Fortunately, I am happy to report I delivered a healthy 7 pounds 6 ounces baby girl. She arrived naturally in the comfort of my home with no complications. It all started with me taking back the control.

Ok! Now you understand why eating clean and detoxifying your body is important. However, we still need proper exercise. It really goes hand and hand. You have to train dirty as well as eat clean.

Train dirty? Sounds gross right? I promise you it is not that bad. If you dedicate 30 minutes a day with a high impact routine, you will definitely see the results you want. Yes, you can still lose weight without exercising. But are you happy with being content? I don't know about you, but I don't wake up every day hoping to be mediocre. I don't want to just get rid of the weight. I want to add definition to my body, I want to build endurance, and I want to look great!

Benefits of working out:

- Better Sleep
- Reduces Stress
- Energy Boost
- Increase Strength
- Improve Self-Confidence
- Sharpens Memory
- Increases Sex Drive
- Reduces Risk of Chronic Diseases

I put together a routine for the next 21 days that is very simple and easy to do. You can do this at home, a park, or at the gym. No weights are needed with this routine. If you wanted to add weights with this program, you most certainly can.

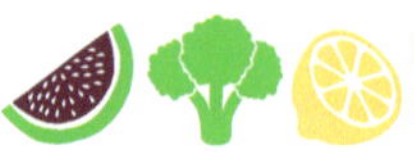

<u>7 TIPS BEFORE YOU GET STARTED</u>

1. **Plan Ahead-** This tip is the most important tip. Prepare yourself for the next 21 days. You can break it down into 3 weeks (7 days a week for next 3 weeks=21 days). These means shop for the week. Know what you want to prepare and plan your schedule. You can mix and match the recipes or eat the same thing for the next 21 days. Whatever it is you do, just be prepared.

2. **Stay Hydrated-** The goal is to drink 1 liter a day of water. You can add apple cider vinegar, honey, and lemon to your water as well. This will help with burning the fat. If you add cayenne pepper it will help with the circulation of the blood. Herbal teas are also a good source of fluid. I recommend green tea, ginger tea, and mint tea. They are all good for blood circulation and fat burning.

3. **Whole Foods only-** For next 21 days you will not consume processed foods, meats, dairy, animal products, liquor, coffee, refined carbs, caffeinated drinks, etc.

4. **Stay Close to a Bathroom-** Take this advice from my own personal experience. If you are not use to going on a regular basis…this will definitely help you do that. Also have baby wipes with you to keep yourself feeling fresh.

5. **Pack Snacks-** This goes back to meal prepping. Snacks are allowed but only raw nuts, fruits (preferably high in water content like watermelon), and raw veggies. This will be a staple in your food palate.

6. **Daily Affirmation-** Repeat every day **"I AM HAPPY & HEALTHY. I AM COMMITED TO MY SUCCESS."** Affirmations will help you stay focus. It is better to repeat in front of the mirror to remind yourself how great you are!

7. **Follow me on Instagram: @melonated and take before and after pictures and send to** melonated365@gmail.com **or tag me in a post.**

ON YOUR MARK, GET SET, READY, GO!

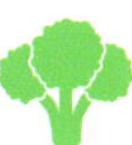

PART I: EAT CLEAN

"Let food be thy medicine and medicine be thy food." -Hippocrates

Every day, for next 21 days, your meals will consist of smoothies, soups, salads, juice, and occasional "heavy meal". Most of your meals are a form of liquid. The reasoning behind this is, I want you to constantly flush your system and get rid of any toxins. My "heavier meals" will consist of brown rice, gluten free pasta, potatoes, wraps, etc. I don't want you to feel like you are starving, however I want you to realize the importance of consuming less animal protein and processed foods.

You may snack in between. Remember your snack will be a choice of fruits, raw veggies, or raw nuts. Do not forget to stay hydrated by drinking 1 liter of water a day. The water will help flush your system throughout the course of your day. Furthermore, all your meals will have been eaten before 7pm each day. If you do not have a juicer, just make an extra smoothie.

LEAN, MEAN, VEGGIE MACHINE.

It is very important to have a balance healthy way of living. The Eat Clean and Train Dirty plan is not about starving yourself or try to convert you into becoming a vegan. It is about starting new healthy habits. Most people are concerned about protein and how they are going to get the right amount over the course of 21 days. The answer is VEGETABLES! There are plenty of vegetables out there that are very high in protein. Also I find it quiet funny that we as human beings, once we start trying to do something a little bit different, we start to think of ways of why it would not work. Just think about it. When you are ordering from Mc Donald's or your favorite restaurant, are you asking the person who is servicing you "how many grams of protein this meal has?" The answer is NO!

Also keep in mind cows and chickens are vegetarians, so where do they get there protein from? You might as well go straight to the source.

<u>15 Highest Protein Vegetables</u>

1. Chickpeas-6 grams
2. Chia Seeds-6 grams
3. Spinach-3 grams
4. Avocado-2 grams
5. Broccoli- 2 grams
6. Lima Beans-7.3 grams
7. Black Beans- 7.6 grams
8. Tofu-8 to 15 grams
9. Tempeh- 16 grams
10. Lentils- 9 grams
11. Asparagus- 2.4 grams
12. Pumpkin Seeds- 5grams
13. Kale-2.5 per cup
14. Artichoke- 4 grams
15. Edamame- 6grams

Vegetables bring an important balance to your health. It helps reduce risks of a lot of chronic diseases. Whereas animal protein are highly like to cause chronic diseases. According to Harvard T.H. Chan School of Public Health," *The higher the average daily intake of fruits and vegetables, the lower the chances of developing cardiovascular disease. Compared with those in the lowest category of fruit and vegetable intake (less than 1.5 servings a day), those who averaged 8 or more servings a day were 30 percent less likely to have had a heart attack or stroke.*"

Green vegetables are full of fiber and vitamins. They can decrease cholesterol levels and prevent cell damaging. Studies shows dark leafy greens such as kale, spinach, broccoli, and bok choy contains an abundance of carotenoids-antioxidants. This protects the cells and blocks the early stages of cancer. Consuming dark leafy greens on a daily basis is very vital to a balance diet. It also regulates the digestive system helps in weight management and bowel health.

****Important Tip***

When purchasing your greens vegetables, please do not buy 21 DAYS WORTH. Greens can go bad very quickly if not consumed in a timely manner. You showed be restocking on greens at the most every 7 days.

Instagram: @melonated
melonated365@gmail.com

"Progress is impossible without change, and those who cannot change their minds cannot change anything."

-George Bernard Shaw

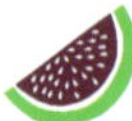

GROCERY HAUL

In this eBook they are a few recipes and everyday items that you will need to go to the grocery store for to be prepared for each week. There is no need to buy the entire list all at once. You can replenish at the as you go along. Your staple foods will be your fruits, greens, and nuts. To sustain you throughout the day, pack a small bag of your favorite fruits, nuts, or veggies, and create a trail mix.

You can shop at your local farmers market or grocery store to obtain these items.

- 1 Bag of red or green apples
- 1 Bag of carrots
- 3 bunches of Kale
- 1 Spring Mix Greens
- 1 Pack of spinach
- 1 Pack of tofu
- 6 Red potatoes
- 1 bunch of bananas
- 1 pack of blue berries
- 1 pack of strawberries
- 1 Pack of Raw almonds, walnuts, cashews, and brazil nut
- Almond Milk (Unsweetened) or your choice of non dairy milk.
- Raw Uncooked Unfiltered Honey or Agave
- Chia Seeds
- Flax Seeds
- 1 Pack of Water (Liter Size)
- Jump Rope (for fitness)
- 1 Pack of Frozen mangos
- 1 Pack frozen strawberries
- 1 Pineapple
- 1 pack of Large celery stalk
- 1 pack of cucumbers
- 2 pieces of ginger root
- Maca
- 2 Avocado (Per Week)
- 1 can of Coconut Milk
- Curry Powder

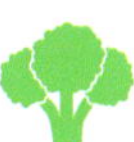

- 1 pack of cucumbers
- Brown rice (Jasmine brown rice is easier to cook)
- 1 Pack of lentils
- 1pack of red kidney beans/black beans
- 1 pack of gluten-free penne pasta
- 1 pack of gluten-free linguini pasta
- 1 Pack of organic Vegetable broth
- Olive Oil (Cold Pressed)
- Cayenne pepper
- Garlic powder
- Onion powder
- Organic Apple Juice
- Orange Juice (Not From Concentrate)
- Brown sugar
- Bok choy
- Sweet and sour sauce
- Soy sauce
- BBQ Sauce (preferably natural such as Annie's BBQ)
- Shredded collard greens
- Red onion/yellow onion
- Vegan Mayonnaise (preferably Vegenaise or Hellmann's Vegan Mayonnaise)
- Brown Mushrooms
- Pink Sea Salt or Morton's Nature's seasoning.

Now that you have gotten your list for the week, you are ready to begin.

I have broken down the 21 days into 3 weeks. The most important thing to remember is to keep it simple. You do not need to overwhelm yourself with countless recipes and fitness routines. Just take it week by week. If you plan ahead, it will help you get through this program with ease. You can also implement the same meals each week to make it less complicated.

WHERE DID THE TIME GO?

As a mom of an energetic 2 year old, a wife, and full-time entrepreneur or what I like to call it, mompreneur, time EVERYTHING. It is really beneficial to me to create time for things that are important for my health and well being. Some of you may argue, "Well I work a 9-5 and I am a single parent." Listen you can still be in a relationship and still be a single parent. Furthermore, working for yourself requires you to put in more time past the traditional 8 hour routine. You need to create time for the things that are important to your life. Therefore, health and wellness should be at the top of your list.

 Find time to fit in your fitness routine each day. Early mornings will be the best time to work out, even if it is for 30 minutes a day. In my experience, morning workouts keep you energized and excited. You also can get a lot more done when you start earlier.

If the mornings are not in your favor, the next best thing will be between the hours of 7pm-8pm. By this time you have already finished your last meal and burning calories will be a lot more effective.

A typical schedule will be:

SUN	MON	TUE	WED	THUR	FRI	SAT
REST DAY	5AM-6AM Workout	5AM-6AM Workout	5AM-6AM Workout	5AM-6AM Workout	REST DAY	7:00AM-7:30AM Breakfast
7:00-8:00am Breakfast	7:30-8am Breakfast	7:30-8am Breakfast	7:30-8am Breakfast	7:30-8am Breakfast	7:30-8am Breakfast	8:30-9:30am Workout
Lunch 12-1	Lunch 12-1	Lunch 12-1	Lunch 12-1	Lunch 12-1	Lunch 12-1	Lunch 12-1
Snack 2pm-3pm	Snack 2pm-3pm	Snack 2pm-3pm	Snack 2pm-3pm	Snack 2pm-3pm	Snack 2pm-3pm	Snack 2pm-3pm
Dinner 5pm-6pm	Dinner 5pm-6pm	Dinner 5pm-6pm	Dinner 5pm-6pm	Dinner 5pm-6pm	Dinner 5pm-6pm	Dinner 5pm-6pm

"You can make up whatever it is that you want, just don't make up excuses"-Gina Mondesir

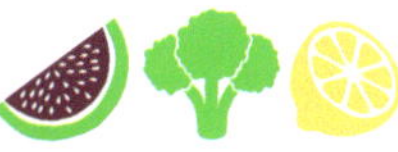

Now let's get ready to eat clean!

WEEK1:

Breakfast: Peanut Punch Smoothie (24oz drink)

    3 scoops of raw peanut butter

    3 cups of Almond milk

    2 tablespoons of Chia seeds

    1 whole banana

    1 tablespoon of Maca

    2 tablespoons of raw uncooked unfiltered honey (or agave)

Add ice and blend until it is smooth!

Lunch: Island Breeze Smoothie (16 oz drink)

    1 cup of frozen mango

    1 cup of frozen strawberries

    2 cups of spinach

    1 cup of Orange Juice (Simply Orange juice)

    1cup of unsweetened Almond milk

    Blend until it is smooth!

Snack: Your choice of a fruit, raw veggies, or raw nuts (It can be a combination of all three)

Drink your water

Dinner: Avocado Corn Salad

    Spring mix greens

    Chopped Red onions

    Chopped Bell peppers

Instagram: @melonated
melonated365@gmail.com

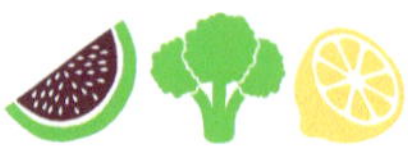

Ripe cherry tomatoes

1 cup of loose kernel corn

Mix with your favorite dressing (Stay away from dressing that has dairy)

*****Drink all your water before bed*****

WEEK 2

Breakfast: Avocado & Banana Smoothie (24 oz)

    1 whole banana

    Half of ripe avocado

    3 cups of almond milk

    1 table spoon of Chia seeds

    1 tablespoon of ground flax seeds

    2 tablespoon of raw uncooked unfiltered honey (or agave)

Add ice. Blend until it is smooth!

Lunch: Green Goodness (12-16 oz)

    3 apples

    2 bunch of Kale

    3 cups of spinach

    4 celery stalk

    2 cucumbers

Snack: Your choice of a fruit, raw veggies, or raw nuts (It can be a combination of all three)

*****Drink your water*****

Dinner: Lentil Soup

    2 cups of dry lentils

    ½ a cup chopped red onion

    1 chopped yellow onion

Instagram: @melonated
melonated365@gmail.com

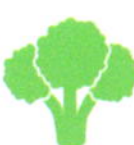

2 chopped carrots

2 chopped celery stalk

3 clove garlic minced

4 cups of vegetable broth (Organic)

4 cups of water

1 chopped tomato

3 table spoon of marinara sauce

1 cup of spinach

¼ olive oil

Add garlic powder, onion powder, salt, and pepper to taste.

Step 1: In a large pot, heat oil over medium heat. Add celery, carrots, garlic, tomato, red onion, yellow onion; Stir in marinara sauce. Add salt and pepper. Sauté for 1 minute.

Step 2: Stir in lentils, add vegetable broth and water. Bring to a boil. Reduce heat. Let it simmer for an hour. Add spinach, garlic powder, onion powder, salt and pepper to taste. Bon Appétit!

*****Drink your water before bed*****

WEEK 3

Breakfast: KALE YEAH SMOOTHIE (24oz)

3 cups of raw apple juice (Simply Apple Juice)

4 cups of kale

1 whole banana

1 cup of frozen strawberries

1 table spoon chia seed

3 tablespoon of agave (raw honey uncooked unfiltered)

Add ice. Blend until it is smooth

Lunch: (Banana Mango Bliss)

1 frozen banana

2 cups of frozen mango

2 tablespoon of hemp seed

Add ice. Blend until it is smooth!

Snack: Your choice of a fruit, raw veggies, or raw nuts (It can be a combination of all three)

*****Drink your water*****

Dinner: Coconut Curry Tofu Soup

1pkg of firm tofu

2 cup of coconut milk

1 tbsp of cayenne pepper

1 tbsp of curry powder

½ cup of tomatoes sauce

½ cup of diced tomatoes

2 cups of chopped onions

2 cups of chopped bell peppers

1 cup of scallions

½ cup of chopped garlic

1 pkg of mix vegetables

2 cups of vegetable broth

½ cup of lima beans

½ cup of corn

Step 1: First heat up the oil in the deep fryer. If you don't have a deep fryer, you can use a regular pot to fry the tofu.

Step 2: Then cut the block of tofu into medium-squared shapes. While the oil is hot; place the tofu into the deep fryer. Cook until the tofu is a golden brown color.

Step 3: In a skillet, sauté the corn, lima beans, chopped onions, chopped bell peppers, and chopped garlic until it is lightly browned. Stir in tomato sauce.

Step 4: Mix in Tofu, curry powder, cayenne pepper, and coconut milk.

Step 5: Add vegetable broth. Allow the Coconut Curry Tofu Soup to simmer for 10 minutes

Bon appétit!

*****Drink your water before bed*****

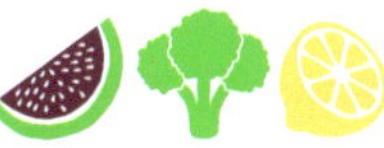

Bonus Recipe Ideas

<u>Smoothies</u>

- **Summer Sunset Smoothie (24 oz)**

   1 cup of frozen mango
   1 cup of pineapple
   1 cup of chopped strawberries
   1/2 cup of frozen grapes
   ½ cup of frozen papaya
   3 cups of 100% natural coconut water

 Place all the above ingredients into a blender with ice. Blend until smooth.
Adjust sweetness according to taste and pour into a cup!

- **Pineapple Splash Spice (24oz)**

   ¼ cup of chopped ginger
   1 cup of pineapple
   2 cup of Natural Lemonade
   1 cup of water
   1 cup of spinach
   2 tbsp of agave
   ½ cup of frozen grapes

Place all the above ingredients into a blender with ice. Blend until smooth.
Adjust sweetness according to taste and pour into a cup!
Enjoy a healthy way of living!

<u>Juices</u>

- **Carrot Passion Juice**
   6 large carrots halved

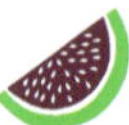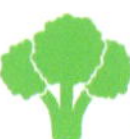

1 orange peeled

1 grape fruit peeled

3 celery stalk

1 tea spoon of ground turmeric

Get Right Ginger Juice

4 green apples

6 large carrots

4 tbsp of ginger

1 bunch of kale

<u>Meals</u>

- **Kale Pasta Salad**

  2 cups of raw Kale

  2 cups Gluten-free penne pasta

  1 cup of chopped red onion

  ½ cup of green onion

  1 diced tomato

  2 tbsp of vegan mayonnaise

  1 cup of arugula

  Salt & pepper to taste

Step 1: Boil pasta according to package.

Step 2: In a desired bowl mix in kale, red onion, green onion, tomato, and arugula. Stir in pasta and mayo. Add salt and pepper

Bon Appétit!

- **Minestrone Soup**

  2 cups of raw red kidney beans (not in can)

  2 stalk of celery chopped

  6 cups of vegetable broth

  2 cups of water

  2 cups of diced tomatoes

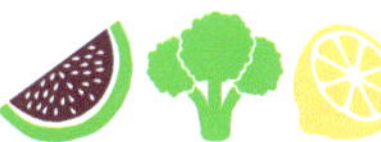

1 chopped onion
1 cup diced carrots
1 cup of elbow pasta (gluten free)
1 cup of fresh chopped basil
1 table spoon of oregano
2 tablespoon of olive oil
3 tablespoon of marinara sauce
Garlic powder, onion powder, Salt & Pepper to taste

Step 1: First boil kidney beans according to package or until tender.
Step 2: In a separate large pot, heat olive oil over medium heat. Add onion, carrots, celery, tomatoes, and kidney beans. Stir marinara sauce. Combine seasoning and sauté for 2 minutes.
Step 3: Mix in vegetable broth and add water. Stir in pasta. Let it simmer for 15 minutes. Add basil and oregano. Finish off with salt and pepper to taste.
Bon Appétit!

- **Berry Spinach Salad**
  1 cup of chopped strawberries
  ½ cup of sliced raw almonds
  3 cups of spinach
  ½ cup of chopped onions
  ½ cup of raisins
  Mix in strawberry vinaigrette dressing

*****If you have an idea for a recipe, you are more than welcome to incorporate into this program. As long as it is a soup, salad, smoothie, or juice.*****
Enjoy a healthy way of living!

HEAVY MEALS RECIPIES

This section is for those of you who want little bit more and like the idea of feeling full. Coming from a Caribbean background, this has always been my challenge when I started to create healthier eating habitats. This led me to begin experimenting with some of my favorite recipes and adding a holistic twist. You can easily take any of these recipes and added to your lunch or dinner meal option for the week or that day. Remember do not get overwhelmed with these recipes.I want you to focus on your goal of cleansing your body.

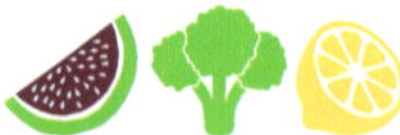

My goal for you is to create new habits and for my readers to adopt the idea to "Eat for nutrition and not for taste."

- **Island Brown Rice and Mushroom Collard Greens**

Ingredients:
- 2 cups of Brown Rice
- 1 cup of chopped red onion
- 1 cup yellow onion
- 3 table spoons of minced garlic
- 2 cups of brown mushrooms
- 4 cups of shredded collard greens
- 2 cups of black beans
- 1 cup of green/red bell peppers
- 2 tbsp. tomato sauce
- 1 cup of Olive oil
- 3 cups of water
- 1 cup of diced tomatoes

Step 1: Boil black beans according to package
Step 2: Add oil to pot and place on medium heat. Allow the oil to heat up no more than 2 minutes. Then place chopped yellow onions and minced garlic to the pot. Cook it until it is golden brown. Mix in black beans and tomato sauce. Sprinkle Morton's seasoning (Or any seasoning you prefer) to the beans. Let it cook for 2 minutes. Then add water to the pot. Allow the water to boil for 5 minutes. Stir in brown rice, keep stove on medium heat and let it cook for 30-35 minutes.
Step 3: Add oil to the pot and place over medium heat. Add mushrooms, bell peppers, and diced tomatoes. Cook it for 5 minutes. Mix in collard greens, red onion, and add seasoning to taste. Place heat low. Let it simmer for 10 minutes. You may add ½ cup of water or vegan butter so veggies won't stick to pot. Enjoy a healthy way of living.

Important Tip

You may cook rice according to package. Also choose how much or how little you want to make.

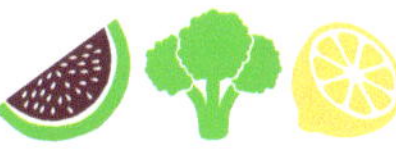

Sautee Veggies and Vegan Potato Salad

Ingredients:

    Vegetable oil
    1 cup of chopped yellow onion
    1 chopped bell peppers
    2 Chopped unpeeled red potato
    Vegan Mayonnaise
    1 cup of green onion
    2 cups broccoli
    2 Cups of chopped carrots
    1 cup of Bok Choy
    1 cup of brown mushrooms
    1 cup of cooked loose corn
    Salt and pepper
    Mustard (Optional)
    3 table spoon of BBQ Sauce (Annie's BBQ sauce recommended)
    1 cup soy sauce
    Garlic powder, Onion powder
    Salt
    Pepper
    1 cup of water.

Step 1: Boil red potatoes for 15 minutes until tender. Let it cool down for 5-7 minutes.

Step 2: Add oil to pot and place over medium heat. Place green onion and chopped garlic to the pot. Cook until it is golden brown. Mix in the bok choy, carrots, broccoli, corn, and mushroom. Then add soy sauce, BBQ sauce, and water. Season this with salt, pepper, garlic powder, and onion powder. Let this cook for 10 minutes.

Step: Place red Potatoes in bowl. Mix in onions, bell peppers, mayonnaise, mustard, salt, and pepper. Stir together until it is even on all sides.

Voilà! Enjoy a healthy way of living.

Important Tip

It is very important to season to your liking. You can also add, or take away any of the veggies to customize this to you.

PART II: TRAIN DIRTY

"Take care of your body. It's the only place you have to live." *~Jim Rohn*

Following your daily routine of eating clean for the next 21 days, you are going to incorporate a fitness routine. This will help you get things in your body circulating, boost energy, and build confidence. These simple exercises can be done at home, the park, or a gym. Weights are not necessary. However if you want to add weights, you are more than welcome too!

Each day you will build on the next exercise.

Remember to push yourself to the best of you ability. If you get frustrated, repeat your daily affirmations to yourself: *"I am happy and healthy. I am committed to my success."*

<u>**Now let's get ready to train dirty!**</u>

21 DAY FITNESS GUIDE

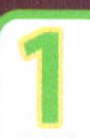

1

40 Squats
10 Crunches
20 Lunges
10 Push Ups
2 mins. Jump Rope

2

45 Squats
15 Crunches
25Lunges
10 Push Ups
2 mins. Jump Rope

3

55 Squats
15 Crunches
30 Lunges
12 Push Ups
4 mins. Jump Rope

4

60 Squats
20 Crunches
35 Lunges
15 Push Ups
4 mins. Jump Rope

5	6	7	8
REST TODAY YOU DESERVE IT!	65 Squats 25 Crunches 35 Lunges 15 Push Ups 6 mins. Jump Rope	70 Squats 25 Crunches 40 Lunges 15 Push Ups 6 mins. Jump Rope	80 Squats 30 Crunches 45 Lunges 20 Push Ups 8 mins. Jump Rope
9	**10**	**11**	**12**
REST TODAY YOU DESERVE IT!	85 Squats 35 Crunches 45 Lunges 22 Push Ups 8 mins. Jump Rope	90 Squats 35 Crunches 50 Lunges 22 Push Ups 10 mins. Jump Rope	95 Squats 40 Crunches 50 Lunges 25 Push Ups 10 mins. Jump Rope
13	**14**	**15**	**16**
REST TODAY YOU DESERVE IT!	100 Squats 40 Crunches 55 Lunges 25 Push Ups 2 mins. Jump Rope	100 Squats 45 Crunches 60 Lunges 30 Push Ups 4 mins. Jump Rope	105 Squats 45 Crunches 60 Lunges 30 Push Ups 4 mins. Jump Rope

17	**18**	**19**	**20**
110 Squats	**REST**	115 Squats	120 Squats
50 Crunches	**TODAY**	55 Crunches	60 Crunches
60 Lunges	**YOU DESERVE IT!**	65 Lunges	70 Lunges
30 Push Ups		35 Push Ups	40 Push Ups
4 mins. Jump Rope		6 mins. Jump Rope	10 mins. Jump Rope

DAY 21
YOU MADE IT!

Instagram: @melonated
melonated365@gmail.com

The Finish Line

"No one has a problem with the first mile of a journey. Even an infant could do fine for a while. But it isn't the start that matters. It's the finish line."

— Julien Smith,

Give yourself a round of applause! You deserve a standing ovation. Statistic says that only 2% of people ever finish what they started. Why do you think that is? Is it fear of failure or fear of success? I think it is a little bit of both. We as humans are afraid of how great we can become once we live up to our fullest potential.

I know sometimes I have those fears. Nevertheless, I turn my fears into fuel. The very thing that's scares me is the same thing that motivates me. Seems crazy right?

We should live everyday being the best versions of ourselves. Yes, not every day is a good day. However, every day is an opportunity to make it great. And if nobody told you this during your 21 day journey of eating clean and training dirty, I AM PROUD OF YOU! I am proud that you saw it through until the end, I am proud that you were fearless throughout the process, and I am proud that you became a living example of your new lifestyle.

Welcome to a better way of living!

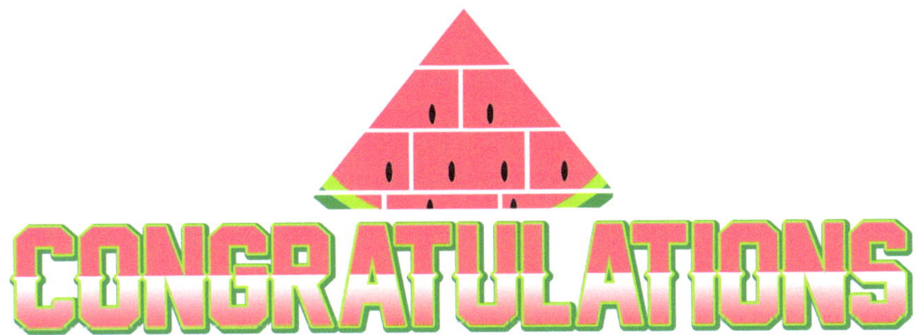